Managing Climate Change Consequences

And Other Critical Issues

Dr. ANDREA SCARSI

DEDICATED

To Mother Earth and All Souls She's Carrying

CONTENTS

DR. ANDREA SCARSI

NOTE OF THE AUTHOR

The Author strived to be accurate and complete when creating this book. Nevertheless, he affirms that the contents expressed in it are solely the result of his knowledge, experience, and competence in the considered discipline and does not guarantee and declare at any time that these are absolute and unequivocal.

While he made all attempts to verify the information in this publication, he assumes no responsibility for errors, omissions, different interpretations, or experimentations of the subject matter herein.

Any perceived slights of specific persons, peoples, companies, or organizations are unintentional.

There are no guarantees of performed results or income made in self-help books and manuals, as one expects. Readers must rely on their judgment about any single circumstance and act accordingly.

This book does not pretend to be an official medical, dietetic, psychological, religious, legal, commercial, accounting, or financial professional source. The Readers must seek the services of competent professionals in all the abovementioned fields.

Enjoy your practice.

DR. ANDREA SCARSI

DESCRIPTION

Floods, earthquakes, heatwaves, landslides, wildfires, blackouts, terrorism, and so on are all happening now! If we don't know how to deal with them and how to get ready, we run the risk of hopelessness and despair for our loved ones and us. But knowledge is power, and there's always something we can do. This survival manual is designed for those who want to understand the most common emergencies and catastrophes caused by natural phenomena or human activities.

Natural calamities can, indeed, strike at any time, and this can be said with certainty because those of us who have already completed our first half-century of age have personally experienced many of these events in our lifetime. The unpredictability of these situations is a stark reminder that vigilance is key; Gaia rarely warns us when it will release heavy rains, incredible hurricanes, shocking earthquakes, lightning storms, or historical volcanic eruptions. She goes on her way and carries us.

The long list of recent tornadoes, tsunamis, avalanches, and earthquakes around the world is a sobering reminder for all and all of us never to take nature for granted and always to know what to do in case Gaia, for reasons of its own, is ready to strike again. We should look for specific steps to prepare ourselves, our families, friends, and acquaintances if a massive event, natural or artificial, happens. This vigilance and readiness are critical to our survival, keeping us alert and prepared for any eventuality.

Never take lightly any natural upheavals, and never consider them with the fatality and cynicism of the inevitable, irreparable eventualities to which we can only helplessly surrender; they manifest, and we must be ready and willing to limit or even prevent any damage, thanks to the experience acquired by our species.

When we prepare ourselves as well as possible, we ride the disasters, which Gaia wants. She wants us to learn to know her. This book results from a joint effort of consciousness to remain awake, alert, and ready. It is specialized research to be shared, emphasizing the need for a collective responsibility, which ensures that even in the most intense scenes, the ones we love and our fellowmen in toto are safe and damages scarce or limited to the very minimum.

FLOOD

Floods are widespread in tropical countries, but that doesn't mean that temperate and wintry countries don't experience flooding, one of the most common natural disasters in various parts of the world. It won't change anytime soon, so we'd best be prepared for this type of emergency.

There are generally two kinds of floods.

The first type of flood develops over a long period due to continuous rain. Preparing for this type of flooding is usually easier because you can gather your emergency supplies as you monitor the rising waters around the neighborhood.

The second type of flooding, flash flood, is more sudden. Flash floods happen within a few minutes, and neighborhoods can submerge without warning. Flash floods can occur in the following situations:

Excessive rainfall over a long period

Structural or operational dam problems

Ice jam breakage

An overflow in natural bodies of water, such as rivers.

Street drains that cannot handle the water coming in from excessive rainfall.

While regular floods carry some debris, flash floods are doubly dangerous because flash flood waters often move rocks and mud. Imagine a massive wave of muddy and rocky water heading toward your neighborhood.

In Southeast Asian countries, flash floods have been known to decimate whole communities in hours. Little can be done if the victims of flash floods have modest or no knowledge of how to act during a natural disaster. While some cities are relatively safe from flooding, one can never know. Be extra alert if you live in a low-lying area near any body of water since even a pond can cause massive flooding during a torrential downpour.

Many people have yet to experience a devastating flood — and that's good. Suppose you have never experienced it in your lifetime. In that case, it means that you live in a flood-protected area or your local government is doing everything possible to prevent flooding, even during the worst downpours.

However, that doesn't mean you won't have to know how to act during a flood. Not necessarily; waves can take place anywhere because every area in every country experiences changes in topography. Soil moves, though very slowly, and over time, this will impact how flood-proof a city or town is.

Ask if you need clarification on how safe your neighborhood is from flooding. Indeed, some old-timers in your area may or may not have experienced flooding some years ago. Suppose flooding has occurred in your neighborhood, even if it was ten years ago. In that case, your community will probably experience flooding again if a sufficient number of factors come into play.

FLOOD FACTS

Hurricanes are more devastating than tropical storms because they carry more wind force, debris, and floodwater. Both tropical storms and hurricanes can cause flooding, and both can cause massive property damage. Coastal areas are more likely to experience the full extent of hurricanes; if you live in such a place, you may already be aware of the swiftness of the floods that intense storms can bring.

Melting snow and ice during spring can cause flooding if you live near natural bodies of water such as ponds and streams. The land doesn't absorb all that melted snow since everything freezes during winter, including the soil. Frozen soil is less absorbent, caused by particles stuck together and allowing very little moisture to seep through.

Northern or southern regions, according to the hemisphere, are at high risk for flooding due to excessive rainfall. Excess rainfall is often the result of a coupled oceanic-atmospheric phenomenon, which affects different countries, if not in the present, even all.

Wildfires can also increase the risk of flooding in certain areas. Regions that have frequent fires tend to develop strong mudflows during torrential downpours, which directly impact surrounding towns and cities.

MONITOR FLOODING IN YOUR AREA

When a flood watch has been announced, there's a high probability of flooding. Listen to your radio or local news channel to monitor the progression of the hurricane, storm, or heavy downpour.

That also applies to a flash flood watch. If a flash flood watch has been announced, assume the worst and prepare your emergency kit if you must evacuate your home.

When a local news station announces a flood warning or flash flood warning, prepare to leave your home in case a lot of water is coming into your neighborhood.

The high-level ground is your only absolute protection from floods. Do not attempt to face severe floods by staying home – you will lose to Mother Nature because water can flood even the most fortified of houses.

DRIVING IN FLOODED AREAS

If you find yourself driving through flooded roads and a flooded neighborhood, here are some tips to keep you safe.

Knowing the height of the flood is of utmost importance if you want to try to drive through a flooded area. If you estimate six inches of floodwater, be aware that this much water can probably penetrate the inside of your car and mess with your vehicle's brake system and transmission.

Driving through six inches of water will probably leave you wet and stranded in a flooded area unless you drive a highly capable four-wheel drive or a flatbed truck. If more water comes, more water will penetrate your car, causing additional hazards for you and your passengers.

An area with at least twelve inches of flood water will automatically stall and float a vehicle; don't try to drive through such areas. You will be stranded, and if the water goes up again, your car will be carried away by the current until the flood water finally subsides.

The best driving advice anyone can give you when facing a flooded road is not driving through it. Find another way if possible. If you can't, wait until the flood subsides. It's rarely worth the risk anyway.

Your intentions may be correct (i.e., driving home to your family during a stormy night), but if there's a flood, you might get stalled halfway through, and your family will have additional problems.

If a road has been barricaded recently due to flooding, don't try to drive around it. Roadblocks were installed to prevent people from being stalled or even floated away by floodwaters.

Driving at night through flood roads can be extremely dangerous. If you have to drive through floodwater, use your brightest lights and drive slowly so you can spot potential dangers on the road, such as floating tree branches and other debris. Also, it's extra challenging to evaluate the depth of a flood at night; what may look like four inches of flooding to you may be seven inches of water or more.

DEALING WITH THE FLOOD

If you are at home when the floodwaters arrive, don't panic; there are specific guidelines to help you deal with the watery deluge.

If the power hasn't been knocked out, turn the TV on and monitor the situation through your local news channel. Your radio is also your best friend when receiving updates from a local flood watch.

Has there been an announcement of a possible flash flood? If the answer is yes, seek higher ground immediately. If you have a second or third floor, go upstairs after securing the first one. Do not stay on the first floor if a flash flood is imminent!

If flooding is imminent and you still have time, move all your patio furniture inside the house; if your home has a second or third floor, shift electronic gadgets, large appliances, and other essentials upstairs.

Do this with sufficient time; if not, merely elevate these items on tables, chairs, and your kitchen counters. You can always fix your first floor after the flood. The important thing here is you will be keeping most of your expensive personal possessions safe during the surge while you seek higher ground for yourself.

Water and electricity should be turned off in the event of a flood. Unplug all your electrical appliances, including small items such as radios and fans. Although some of your devices have become submerged in floodwater and cannot be unplugged, don't touch them while they are still immersed in water.

It is dangerous to walk through moving floodwaters, so if you have to do it, ensure the water is no more than five inches deep. Six inches of moving floodwater (with mud and debris) is enough to topple even fit people.

If the water is deep and you must cross it to evacuate or get to your car, find a path across the floodwater with less powerful movement to ensure your safety.

If there are emergency services in your area, you can help the emergency personnel by keeping your family safe and the area clear so that they can move around your neighborhood more easily.

After evacuating, you should only return to your home once it has been announced that the water has dissipated and it is safe to return to your neighborhood. If no such announcements have been made, stay in the designated safe zone/evacuation zone until the authorities give you and everyone else an all-clear signal.

If your car or SUV suddenly stalls while driving away from your flooded house, leave your vehicle and seek higher ground on foot; you will have a better chance of getting help if you walk instead of trying to restart a wet and stalled automobile. Remember: six to twelve inches of floodwater is enough to stall and float most vehicles. So, it doesn't matter if you have a big SUV – water can still stop it.

During a flood, you often find random spots where water has already receded. These spots are not necessarily safe to drive on or walk on because retreated water usually signals soft and weakened soil. Driving through such areas may be dangerous.

Beware of electrically charged floodwater. Electrical wires run underground, and some wires may cause floodwater to become electrically charged.

Minimize or avoid submerging any part of your body in floodwater. Floodwater contains not only soil particles (i.e., mud) but also chemicals (such as gasoline) and, in some instances, sewage. Sewage contamination is universal – you do not want to experience wading through sewage-tinged floodwater.

If flooding damages your septic tank or plumbing system, have these serviced soon after the flood.

Turn on the power only once you have deemed the house dry enough. If you turn on the power immediately after the flood, someone might get accidentally electrocuted.

WHEN EARTHQUAKES STRIKE

Earthquakes, like flooding, can occur at any moment. The good thing about today's technology is that seismologists monitor seismic activity daily, so they can broadcast any impending earthquakes should they occur. Earthquakes are natural phenomena. They happen when large sheets of rock under the soil suddenly release accumulated pressure and force.

As a planet, the Earth is always in a state of change. There are several layers of rock under the soil that we know so well; over time, shifts occur in these rock layers, and when the pressure has to be released, the ground that we walk on can shake so fiercely that buildings, roads, and bridges crumble and collapse.

Countries like Japan are only too familiar with the destructive power of earthquakes. We can never know precisely when a powerful earthquake will strike a town or city, so it is best to be prepared for its sudden manifestation.

Again, if you have never experienced such an occurrence before, don't rest easy – because, according to studies, 45 states are at moderate risk for earthquakes in the United States. Though this phenomenon has historically been associated with the West Coast, facts show that other states are equally at risk.

If a possible earthquake has been announced in your area, you must start preparing for the potential disaster.

Make sure you have an emergency kit ready. We'll discuss emergency kits and emergency supplies at the end of the book.

Shelves and other wooden furniture should be secured to prevent them from toppling during the earthquake.

Heavy objects should be placed as close as possible to floor level. Those heavy items will most likely fall during a quake, which can be dangerous to you and your family. Imagine vases and big books falling around you; earthquakes can easily affect your home.

If you have frames and other hanging decorations near couches, remove them immediately and place them near the floor level, away from beds, seats, couches, etc.

Lighting fixtures should also be secured and braced during an earthquake. Remove the light bulbs if you don't have to brace your accessories at home. It's one thing to clean up fallen fixtures – it's entirely different when you clean up shattered and powdered light bulbs. The dust from shattered light bulbs is poisonous – cover your nose and mouth if you have to clean up stuff like this.

Furniture and large appliances should be fastened or bolted to the floor. Bolting down large appliances is considered a best practice because it prevents the earthquake from toppling your expensive devices. However, if this is not an option, you can strap them to the wall. Before an earthquake, you should obtain the fasteners and straps/ropes.

Most houses, especially those ten years old or older, have minor structural problems, such as cracks in the walls and the foundation. Small cracks in the foundation can become massive fissures during an earthquake.

If you're aware that your house has such defects, it is best to have them repaired as soon as possible by a professional. A strong earthquake can quickly destroy a tiny home in a neighborhood near the epicenter.

Perform regular checks of your home's foundation. It is a good practice to check the foundation every two to three months.

Most homes have a reasonably significant supply of insecticides and other household chemicals. These chemicals must be stored securely in a bolted-down cabinet that can be closed with a latch or lock during an earthquake. Remember the DCH code during an earthquake: D (Drop), C (Cover), & H (Hold On).

EARTHQUAKE FACTS

Earthquakes usually have aftershocks, a series of mini earthquakes that follow the main quake. These mini-earthquakes always have lower intensity, but they can be just as disruptive, especially when people scramble to pick up toppled stuff after the main quake. It's hard to get a stable footing when there are several aftershocks after the main earthquake, so be careful.

A fault refers to the crack in the plates of rock underground. Even the slightest movement can result in an earthquake. In massive earthquakes, the movement may reach up to several yards. The longer the move, the more vigorous the quake.

It is important to understand how earthquake magnitude is measured. The most commonly used system is the Richter scale, which measures the intensity of earthquakes on a scale of 2 to 10.

Less than 2 = these are classified as microearthquakes; people don't feel these, but they can be measured by special seismic equipment.

2 – 2.9 = micro earthquakes.

3 – 3.9 = minor earthquakes that people feel but rarely cause property damage.

4 – 4.9 = Ground movement can be felt indoors; it is unlikely that earthquakes will cause any massive damage within this range.

5 – 5.9 = a moderate earthquake that may severely damage small and poorly constructed structures. It may also cause minor damage to large and well-built structures.

6 – 6.9 = a strong earthquake that may cause property damage across an area measuring one hundred sixty kilometers from the quake's epicenter.

7 – 7.9 = a major earthquake that can cause significant damage across an area that exceeds one hundred sixty kilometers in measurement.

8 – 8.9 = a great earthquake that may affect an area measuring hundreds of kilometers.

9 – 9.9 = a great earthquake that may affect an area exceeding one thousand kilometers.

More than 10 = a massive earthquake that may destroy vast land areas. No earthquake of this magnitude has yet been recorded by seismologists.

Earthquakes can last from a few seconds to several minutes. The shaking or rocking movement is the ground below, releasing seismic energy transmitted or freed by an even lower layer of the Earth.

Seismic energy can be likened to sound energy – it travels in waves, and if the source continues to give it off, the energy waves will keep coming. The problem with earthquakes is that if the movement below the surface of the Earth is significant, the energy released will also be substantial.

If you can imagine shaking a big bottle of soda, the force building up inside is similar to what's happening underground.

Over time, pressure builds up, and that pressure doesn't dissipate – it has to be released because that's how energy works. Unfortunately, when the power is released, the top layer of the Earth shakes rather violently.

HOW TO ACT DURING AN EARTHQUAKE

There's no time to lose if you feel the ground shaking violently.

Lower yourself immediately (drop) and find the sturdiest cover you can (cover). Desks, tables, and so on are suitable covers during an earthquake. Use any piece of furniture that can protect you from falling debris. Run for the kitchen or home office, as these areas usually have the best earthquake covers.

If you cannot find any suitable cover, go to a corner of the house (one without any frames or cabinetry that may fall on you) and cover your head with your arms. Crouch as low as possible and wait for the earthquake to subside.

Keep everyone crouched on the ground. Don't let anyone run around the house to get cellular phones or gadgets just because of an earthquake. That is dangerous; you can call for help after the earthquake. Emergency services are probably on their way anyway, so there's no need to call them.

The worst thing that could happen to you when you're crouching on the floor is to get hit by falling picture frames, vases, and (heaven forbid) cabinets. It's recommended to seek a corner as far away as possible from items that can fall on you.

However, you should also avoid spots near windows and light fixtures. Windows have glass, and glass can shatter or fall off during a violent earthquake. You can get hit by broken glass or by accessories.

Panic is unnecessary if the earthquake strikes while you are still in bed. Beds are usually placed away from light fixtures and windows (unless yours is right next to a window with several panes of glass) and are considered safe places during an earthquake.

Grab your biggest pillow, place it over your head, and await the earthquake. However, if you are right next to cabinets, shelves, large books, and glass windows, run for the nearest and safest corner and crouch there. Remember to cover your head with your arms. If you can find a better cover, such as a small table, use it to protect yourself from falling debris or items.

Some people think doorways are safe places to wait out an earthquake. They're not. Unless a door has been specifically designed to be sturdy and load-bearing, doorways can collapse, so stay away from them. Pass through doorways only if they are nearby, and you know you can find a safer place to wait out the end of the earthquake.

Many people ask: is it safer to go outside during an earthquake? The answer is no – because so many things can go wrong as you dash for the door. You can get hit by falling light fixtures, furniture, large appliances, and big books on top of shelves.

You can also get injured by tripping over electrical wirings and other stuff displaced during a strong earthquake.

If we examine the earthquake drills used in the United States and other countries, the best practice would be to find the safest corner inside the structure and wait until the earthquake runs its course.

If an earthquake strikes while you are still at work, it's better to stay put than to make a mad dash for the elevators. Ironically, this is the first thing people think to do when working several floors up. Using the elevator during an earthquake is dangerous because those things can easily malfunction.

You can get stranded halfway down, or worse, your elevator might suddenly malfunction and plummet to the ground floor like a dead weight.

And no, jumping before the perceived impact won't make your landing less deadly. The force of several tons of steel and cable is the same even if you jump a split second before impact.

Electrical and automatic systems like alarms (and even sprinklers) can suddenly activate during an earthquake. There is no point in trying to turn off these things, so stay put. Also, power can quickly go out due to fractured power lines, so be prepared to navigate in the dark afterward.

Do not try to locate a flashlight when the power goes out during an earthquake. Stay put and focus on protecting yourself and those around you. Having a cover above your head is essential because if something falls on you and knocks you out, your chances of survival greatly diminish if a massive earthquake hits your city or town.

What if you are outdoors during an earthquake? What should you do? Instinct often tells people to make a run for it, but this is the worst possible thing that you can do because you can trample others who are also making a crazy run for it, and you might end up getting hit by something that has already been toppled by the earthquake.

Just stay put during an earthquake. Move away from others who are running aimlessly to avoid getting trampled yourself. Don't let anyone sway you into 'running with the pack' because the 'pack' doesn't know where it's going.

Move away only if necessary and only if a power or telephone line is nearby. Also, avoid areas with big streetlights, as these can fall over quite easily during an earthquake. If you are driving, park your car away from the natural hazards and wait for the quake to stop.

Your car will serve as an adequate head cover from all falling hazards; it is foolhardy to lock your vehicle and make a run for it. Also, buildings are considered hazardous to cars and pedestrians during an earthquake.

When an earthquake suddenly strikes, wide-open spaces, such as parking lots, are your best friends. Also, don't drive during an earthquake! Stop as soon as you find a suitable spot, and wait for the shocks (and aftershocks) to stop before driving again.

If your roof collapses and you cannot escape, you must stay calm to survive. People who panic rarely survive this type of situation because worrying and anxiety take over so much that they cloud judgment.

Here's what to expect when you are buried by debris.

It will be dark.

Dust and other particles might enter your mouth, eyes, and nostrils.

The air around you might become stale and of poor quality.

You might not be able to hear what's happening outside, and you may not be able to gauge whether or not others are hearing that you are trapped under the debris.

With these in mind, here are some essential pointers.

Never try to light up your surroundings with a match or a lighter. If your building or house collapses, there is a big chance that flammable chemicals, or even gas, are present. You would not want to light a big fire while trapped under debris. If you have a cellular phone or small flashlight with you, use that instead.

Moving about too much can disturb the dust around you, making breathing much harder. Don't place yourself in a situation where you are fighting to breathe because you inhale so much dust with every breath.

You mustn't breathe in large amounts of dust particles while trapped. Use a handkerchief or any cloth to cover your mouth and nose. If you have to use your shirt, use it. Unless it's -5 degrees under the debris, you can survive a little chill. But if you suffocate from the dust, you might become unconscious.

Popular culture has taught people a poor technique when seeking help when a person is trapped under debris: screaming or shouting for help. Do not do this.

You will run out of the air faster if you keep shouting. Shouting is physically taxing, and you will want to preserve your energy for as long as possible because you don't know how long until emergency services come to rescue you.

The ideal signaling tool in this type of situation is the whistle. Without it, you can tap on pipes or stones. The sound may be faint, but emergency personnel are excellent at detecting signs of life.

A faint tapping sound is all they need to start digging. Shout if you hear them, but they can't listen. Only shout once they get to you. Doing so will burn your energy, and you will also inhale nasty dust particles in the process.

DEALING WITH DEADLY HEAT

Heat waves occur in almost every part of the world, and in temperate countries, they can cause serious health problems, especially for people not accustomed to hot weather.

A heat wave occurs when the temperature recorded in a given area far exceeds the average temperature. Excessive heat often comes with excessive humidity, making the air hot and stuffy.

Unaccustomed to excessive heat may experience heat cramps (muscular cramping due to temperature change) and heat exhaustion. Heat exhaustion occurs when the blood supply gets diverted to the skin, and the organs receive less blood and oxygen.

The deadliest result of excessive environmental temperature is heat stroke. The body has a natural temperature control mechanism that keeps the body's temperature at a constant level. This physiological mechanism is essential for survival, as the body requires precise conditions to thrive. If you push it too hard, it will eventually fail.

When a person suffers from a heat stroke, his body's temperature regulation mechanism has stopped or is no longer functioning sufficiently to cool the body down. Brain damage is a real possibility during a heat stroke, so you must get the victim of the heat stroke to a hospital as soon as possible.

MONITORING A HEAT WAVE

Just like earthquakes and floods, authorities and weather bureaus also monitor possible heat waves in certain areas so that people can prepare for excessive heat. When an extreme heat warning is announced, a heat wave is likely in the next 1 to 3 days.

Excessive heat warnings are broadcast when local temperatures reach 110 degrees Fahrenheit (110 degrees Fahrenheit is equivalent to 43 degrees Celsius). This temperature can easily cause heat stroke, so you must monitor temperature changes during this time.

THE BEST PRACTICES DURING HEAT WAVES

We can't prevent the environment from overheating, but we can keep ourselves safe during a heat wave. Here are some best practices to protect you from heat wave-related problems.

Keep track of the heat wave any way you can. Two decades ago, people only had three ways to keep track of the weather – newspaper, radio, and TV. Now, people can monitor the weather constantly on personal computers and cell phones.

Use the technology to monitor any significant changes in the weather – that's one way of maximizing the utility of your smart device, too.

Never leave your children in enclosed spaces, such as your car. Even if the air-conditioning is on, your vehicle is still an enclosed space, and heat can again 'cook' the passengers because the air inside the car can become humid and stuffy.

That applies to pets as well. Your dog may have an excellent way of regulating body temperature, but it can still suffer from a heat stroke.

Your home is your shelter against a heat wave. You are safer in your house than anywhere else. Don't go outdoors unless it is necessary. Direct exposure to the sun is a big no-no when there is a heat wave, as the body can quickly absorb heat from the environment.

If you want your body to stay fresh, situate in an excellent, temperature-controlled location.

If you want to venture out during a heat wave, visit air-conditioned places like the library and the mall so you won't suffer too much in the heat. Locations with circulating air are excellent during heat waves.

If the heat wave lasts for days or weeks, change your diet so your body won't exert extra effort to digest your meals. Lighter meals are a must during heat waves.

Don't use salt tablets; your body doesn't need salt tablets to regulate your hydration. Just drink plenty of water (unless you have a health condition that may worsen with additional fluid intake).

Windows that receive the most sunlight during the afternoon should be covered with drapes to reduce heat from your home. Doors and windows should also be weather-stripped to keep out the heat and to keep the colder air inside the house.

Statistically, people in urban areas experience more prolonged heat waves than those in rural areas. If you live in a highly urbanized district, take the necessary precautions and prepare for a worst-case scenario.

Hydration is necessary to keep oneself healthy during a heat wave. Drinking water cools down the body and prevents dehydration. Drink water even if you feel perfectly fine and hydrated.

The body is poor at detecting hydration levels—you may not feel thirsty until you are partially dehydrated. So, drink fresh, cold water—all your body needs to cool down during a heat wave.

Avoid drinking alcoholic beverages and caffeinated products during a heat wave. Both of these kinds of beverages cause dehydration. Caffeine is a natural diuretic, and people tend to urinate more when they're drinking alcohol.

Don't forget to protect your head from the heat if you work outside. A wide-brim hat offers excellent protection for the head.

Remember to call or text people you know who live alone

and do not have air conditioning installed. They may need your help.

Animals should be observed for signs of heat exhaustion and heat stroke. Call your vet if you think your pet is suffering from the heat.

FIRST-AID MEASURES

Recognizing the symptoms of excessive heat-related health problems is crucial. Here are some tips to help you identify and respond effectively.

When it comes to sunburn, immediate action is key. If you notice the skin is very red and painful, with possible blistering, don't hesitate. Take a bath to remove dirt and oils, and apply sterile dressings to any blisters.

Heat cramping: The subject experiences painful muscular cramps in the abdominal and leg muscles. Excessive sweating is also common. First, bring the subject to a significantly lower temperature location. The heat is causing the cramps; the subject has to rest elsewhere. Perform light stretching on the affected muscles to relieve pain.

Give the subject some cold, fresh water. The subject should drink every quarter of an hour, and small sips of water are okay. If the victim feels like throwing up, don't give him any more water; just let him/her rest. Remember, bringing the patient to the hospital is crucial if his condition worsens.

Heat exhaustion: Subjects experiencing heat exhaustion are often highly sweaty, but their skin will have a rather pale pallor and be nippy to the touch. The pulse rate will be relatively weak. The subject will most likely feel exhausted and nauseated. The subject's body temperature may steadily rise if no first aid is given. The subject must be carried away from the source of excessive heat. They must be brought inside if they work outside (preferably in a room with good air conditioning). Loosen the subject's collar, belt, pants, etc. Constrictive clothing can amplify the effects of heat exhaustion. Give the subject a glass of water to slowly sip every fifteen minutes. If the victim feels like throwing up again, don't give him any more water.

Heat stroke: Victims of heat strokes often have a body temperature exceeding 100 degrees Fahrenheit.

Breathing will be rapid but shallow compared to normal breathing. The patient's skin will most likely be red, though sweating may not be present because the body's temperature control mechanism has already failed.

The first thing that you should do is to call emergency services. Perform first aid after you have made the call. A heat stroke is a dire medical emergency, and the patient may die if no treatment is given. Bring the subject to a fresh location. If the subject is unconscious, carry them there. Remove the subject's clothing to help cool down the body. Give the subject a sponge bath to help lower the body temperature. That has to be done continually until emergency services arrive.

Remember, it's crucial to keep the subject as refreshed and comfortable as possible. Turn on any fans or air-conditioning units you may have in the room. Your continuous care can make a significant difference in the patient's recovery.

WATCH OUT FOR LANDSLIDES

During a typical landslide, a significant amount of debris and mud rolls down the side of a mountain straight toward the flatland – where most houses are built.

If you live near an area where landslides can occur after a torrential downpour, you must ensure that you can protect yourself and your family from the destructive force of debris flow.

Preventive Measures.

If you live in an area with frequent mudflow, you must protect your property from sudden debris flow. You can do this by following these simple preventive measures.

If you build a house or a weekend getaway shack, don't construct it near the side of the mountain or valleys where natural erosion occurs at an accelerated pace. Areas with runoff from bodies of water are also a big no-no.

Be knowledgeable about the history of your land. If you are unsure if your property is in the path of mudflow, ask your local town hall. If your area experienced severe debris flow five or ten years ago, one good downpour will take for that to happen again.

One can never tell whether or not a property will experience a landslide, so it is best to be prepared, even if no landslides have occurred in the past few years.

Add some ground cover to strengthen the soil if your house is built on or near a slope. Vegetation helps slow down erosion, the number one cause of debris flow.

Land bereft of significant vegetation often experiences flash floods and debris flow. That is why denuded land not only harms local wildlife but also hurts people living nearby.

Consider constructing retaining walls around your house to protect your property from landslides.

Retaining walls may not stop all debris flow, but at least your home won't be hit directly by the mud and debris. You will have a barrier around your house, giving you enough time to evacuate if you have to.

You must be aware of several warning signs.

Check your surroundings for any significant changes in the landscape. If the slope of a nearby hill changes after a torrential downpour, that might mean that mud and debris from the nearby hill may already be moving downward. You can also observe areas where runoff water usually passes. Minor landslides may also signal the advent of a bigger and more destructive landslide.

If your home is constructed on a steep slope, changes in the soil might affect your doors and windows. For example, your door may suddenly jam for no reason. If you have good reason to believe this is related to changes in your land, have your house checked by a professional. Jammed windows may also signal a landslide.

Regularly inspect the foundation of your home. Do you see any new cracks forming in the foundation? If so, that may also be a sign of an impending landslide.

Water pipes and electrical lines are commonly installed underground. These utility lines are installed so moisture and soil do not frequently break them.

However, movement underneath the soil can fracture water pipes and cut underground power lines during a landslide. Only two common occurrences can cause the breakage of utility lines – earthquakes and landslides. Either way, you have to be prepared for the coming of a natural disaster.

Some slopes develop unsightly bulges right before a landslide.

Movement underneath the soil can cause water to spring from new cracks in the earth. If you see water erupting from different places, that too may signal the coming of a landslide.

Slopes about to become highly eroded tend to become soft and loose. If your house is built on a steep hill, and you feel the ground shifting down whenever you walk, it's time to check if a landslide is about to occur.

If you suddenly hear smashing boulders and trees being uprooted, a landslide is the most common cause of such noises (if no one is clearing the land).

Landslides won't wait until sunrise to happen. An avalanche can occur in the dead of the night or right before the first rays of the sun emerge in the morning. That's why it is so important to recognize the warning signs so you will be prepared just in case.

SAFETY GUIDELINES DURING A LANDSLIDE

Storms are often accompanied by landslides because of the sheer volume of water the soil absorbs during a torrential downpour. Mudflow channels that are usually stable become unstable because of the excessive rain.

That water has to go somewhere because the soil can't absorb the moisture fast enough. With the help of gravity and erosion, landslides occur in the blink of an eye.

With this in mind, you must be extra vigilant when there is a storm or heavy rain, and you live where landslides have occurred. During a torrential downpour, someone has to stay awake to monitor the situation.

Most landslide-related deaths happen because people were asleep when the landslide took place. You can either stay awake and keep everyone in the house safe or sleep and end up submerged in the debris. As you can see, there is no other viable option here.

If you know that there is a landslide heading toward your home, get out of your home at once. Leave your stuff at home and drive away. Of course, find a path that doesn't cross the way of the debris flow.

If the soil has become too soft, leave your car and run for it. However, you must remember that landslides are fast and can often overtake people on foot. So, if you have to run, run as far as possible from the landslide and avoid all spots/ areas where there is even a small amount of flowing debris.

Living near a natural body of water, like a pond, stream, or river, is excellent. But during storms, these bodies of water can endanger you by increasing the chances of flooding and debris flow.

So, during storms, you must monitor the land's slope and the water level in the nearby body of water.

Fluctuations in water level may mean soil and debris movement somewhere else, and you know what that means: eventually, that debris flow will reach your property, too.

Landslides, like earthquakes, are unpredictable. They can go on for a few minutes, stop, and start again. Stay away from your home during a landslide and wait for the authorities to announce that it's safe to return.

If you go back too early, you risk exposing yourself and your family to peril from another landslide. Remember: eroding soil, mud, and debris can flow ceaselessly after a storm.

There's no telling how much erosion has occurred, so it is best to stay in the evacuation shelter until the landslide is over.

If gas, water, and electrical lines are destroyed during a landslide, call the utility companies as soon as possible so they can repair them the same day.

Check the surrounding area for injured individuals. Unless you are highly trained emergency personnel, it is best to call emergency services so you can tell them where to go. Don't bite off more than you can chew during a disaster.

Replanting trees, shrubs, and other vegetation can help prevent landslides; don't forget to do this after the landslide. Planting more vegetation now may mean that there will be no more landslides in five or ten years.

BEATING WILDFIRES

Every year, more and more new homeowners build or buy homes near woodlands and forests to enjoy nature's beauty. Unfortunately, these beautiful stretches of trees, bushes, and grass can easily catch fire on a hot and dry day.

All it takes is a small fire to ignite a wildfire inferno that can spread for miles before emergency services extinguish it.

Wildfires are incredibly challenging to control because they can spread quickly through the bush with little effort. If the grasslands are dry and the winds regularly blow through the land, the fire can lick across miles of dry land in minutes.

Sometimes, fires start instantaneously because of scorching weather. Other massive wildfires start because of accidents (like in 2007, when a young boy admitted that he had been playing with matches that started a fire that destroyed 38,000 acres of land).

Regardless of the cause, if the wildfire is there, you must deal with it, especially if it's only a few hundred meters away from your house. People die in fires because they don't know what to do once it's already there. We don't want this to happen, so here is a special section dealing with wildfires.

PRE-WILDFIRE PREPARATIONS

Living near forests and grasslands is excellent for the mind and body - but unfortunately, living so close to nature has drawbacks.

Wildfires can start at any moment if you have dry weather. So, if you build a house near a forest, it is best to construct your home so that it won't be feeding any wildfire if it should come in the future.

Fireproof, or fire-resistant, construction materials are a little more expensive than regular lumber, but it's well worth it if you think your home is in the path of a wildfire waiting to happen.

Your landscape directly impacts how quickly a wildfire can get to your house. So, if you want to plant trees and other vegetation, choose the ones that resist fire, such as hardwood trees. This type of vegetation can help slow down advancing wildfires.

Install sufficient smoke alarms throughout the house to warn you of an oncoming wildfire at any time of the day.

These smoke alarms should be tested once every 30 days, and their batteries should be replaced regularly. If you don't replace the batteries regularly, the smoke alarms might not work correctly, which can endanger you and your family.

Invest in two or three large fire extinguishers (ABC fire extinguishers are the best choice). Every person in your household should know how to use them.

So, if your teenager is at home and you're not, your son/ daughter can still put out any small fires at home that may otherwise begin a wildfire.

The ABC classification on fire extinguishers stands for the fire's fuel source.

A – ordinary combustible materials such as paper, textiles, plastics, etc.

B – flammable items such as gasoline.

C – electrical equipment such as television sets, appliances, etc.

An ABC fire extinguisher can quell the fire fed by these fuel sources.

Fire tools like rakes should be readily available; keep them where you can grab one and go within seconds.

Invest in a large and robust ladder that can be used to reach your home's roof.

Investing in fire-resistant window drapes doesn't hurt if you have the funds. If a wildfire reaches your home, the curtains will help slow down the advancing fire, giving you time to escape. These items will also help control the devastation of your home.

In the event of a wildfire, removing items around your house that can easily catch fire is best. The more you can delay the advance of the wildfire, the better.

Place all combustible items in a defensible zone that the fire cannot reach. Call emergency services immediately to inform the authorities that a wildfire has already reached your area.

You will need at least one primary source of water outside your home to effectively combat the fire, should it come. A small pool is excellent, but you can also locate a stream or pond to get water to extinguish the wildfire.

You should also invest in a big water hose long enough to extinguish a fire that may erupt in any part of your house (e.g., roof, ceiling, walls, porch area, etc.).

HANDLING AN ACTUAL WILDFIRE

When you see a wildfire, pick up your mobile phone or landline and call 911. Don't panic – the dispatcher needs to know your exact location and the circumstances of the emergency before being able to respond.

After finishing the call, proceed with the other guidelines. Don't skip this first step because if the wildfire becomes significant, you will need all the help you can get.

A wildfire consumes everything in its path, so if it's heading right for your home, grab your emergency supplies/ kit and arrange for temporary housing somewhere else. It can be your parents' house or a friend's house.

It can be anywhere, as long as it is as far away as possible from your location. Do it if you must stay in a hotel for a few days. The purpose of this relocation is to keep everyone safe. You can proceed with other temporary housing plans later on.

It can get sweltering when there's a wildfire, so don't venture out without protective clothing. Pants and long-sleeved shirts are a must. Wear shoes or boots that will fully protect your feet from the heat.

If you have work gloves, wear those as well to protect your hands from blistering. Your face also requires protection—in the absence of a gas mask (which only a few people have), tie a large handkerchief or shirt over your mouth and nose to protect them from dust particles and superheated gases.

Get all of the fire tools that you can so you can protect your home from the fire. If the fire becomes too large to contain, you should get out of there as soon as possible – drive away or run for it! Fire tools include shovels and lots of plastic buckets to carry water.

Homes have natural vents (living room windows, kitchen windows, doors, basement ventilation, etc.). All of these vents must be closed immediately during a wildfire. The fire can enter your house much faster if you open these vents.

Fuel sources, like propane, should be shut off immediately. It's not enough to turn off your oven and stove—you must also turn the valves that control fuel flow from the containers themselves.

You don't need to leave your house if the wildfire is still a few miles away. But at this point, driving your car near the road would be a good idea.

Close the doors and windows, but leave the key inside (in the ignition, preferably). Turn off the engine and leave your vehicle so you can use it immediately when you spot the fire coming too close to your house.

Important documents, such as birth certificates and religious mementos, should be placed in a portable, fireproof, safe box and carried to the car.

Bring only the documents that you really cannot live without. Leave the other documents because you don't want to pile junk into your car while fleeing a wildfire.

If you have a pool or large tub, place all the stuff that water will not destroy in the container or swimming pool. Of course, you will have to fill the pool with water.

This aims to keep some of your possessions safe from fire. You can safely submerge them in water without damaging porcelain vases and dining wares.

Most of our material possessions are incredibly flammable. Move your stuff away from the windows and doors. Put them in the middle of the floor so fires will touch them last.

All doors and windows should be closed, but don't lock any. If your house does catch fire, firefighters may need to enter your home. If you lock the doors and windows, they will use axes and hammers to get through.

USING YOUR VEHICLE DURING A FIRESTORM

While it's not always recommended, using your vehicle as a temporary bunker during a firestorm can provide significant safety. If you're faced with fleeing a fire on foot or using your car, remember that you'll be safer inside your vehicle.

Here are some tips to keep you safe during a firestorm.

Once you enter the car, all air vents should be closed. Headlights should be turned on. Find a path that doesn't have too much smoke. You should be able to see where you're driving.

You don't want to drive through a raging inferno – your tires will pop, and you will be cooked alive if you drive through the fire. Drive away from a firestorm, not through it.

Stay away from vegetation. It's the vegetation that is catching fire in the first place. Sooner or later, the plants that have not yet burned down will be burned down by the firestorm if the bushes and trees are near the wildfire.

If you are surrounded by fire, stay inside your vehicle! Some smoke may enter, but you are far safer inside than outside. Let the central fire run its course; do not run for it on foot because you will be toasted alive outside.

You may feel air currents buffeting your car—this is normal. Don't worry; gas tanks explode only in the movies. If your vehicle is in good condition and your gas tank is closed and secured, your car is not likely to blow.

Disasters can stem from various sources, not just Mother Nature. From terrorist hazards to technological failures like blackouts, this guide covers a range of potential threats. With this knowledge, you'll be better equipped to handle most disasters. Remember, knowledge is power when it comes to disaster preparedness.

BLACKOUTS

Most cities rarely experience blackouts – but what should you do when the power supply suddenly becomes cut off, and you stand in complete darkness?

Pre-Blackout Preparations.

Have your emergency kit ready.

Conserving energy is one way of directly preventing blackouts. The less power you consume, the more electrical energy you distribute to thousands of households around the city.

Rolling blackouts occur because there isn't enough energy to go around, and electric companies tend to impose these blackouts because people are overusing electrical energy. Yes – there is such a thing as energy overuse in the age of nuclear power.

Fill many plastic bags with water and place them in the freezer or refrigerator. These plastic bags will help keep meats and vegetables fresh if a blackout occurs. Outages can sometimes last for days; meat can quickly go rotten if you don't prepare these chilled/ iced bags in advance.

You must keep freezing containers nearby if you use a medication like insulin. Freezing containers contain special fluids that remain cold even if the refrigerator is off.

Always keep your vehicle's gas tank at least half full. Gas

pumps work by electricity. During a blackout, gas stations without a backup generator may not be able to provide gas to travelers.

Many homes have automatic electric garage doors. These doors may be safe and convenient but become useless during blackouts. Equipping your electric garage doors with manual release levers is a good idea. Manual release levers allow the owner to open and close the garage doors even if there isn't any power.

Ensure you know where the manual release lever is and how to use it during blackouts. You don't want to be stuck at home without handling your car because the garage door won't open.

Some people like using the garage entrance to enter their homes, but this might not be the best route if there's a blackout. So, to ensure you can enter your house during an outage, always carry a spare key with you.

If you use a motorized wheelchair or battery-operated scooter, ensure you have a spare battery (fully charged, of course) so you don't have to worry about being unable to move during the blackout.

BLACKOUT SAFETY GUIDELINES

The following are safety guidelines to use when a blackout is upon you.

Candles are a big no-no during outages because these easily fall over and burn down part of the house. You also cannot depend on live fire (i.e., candles) because these tend to run out fairly quickly. Invest in high-quality LED flashlights and emergency lights instead.

A 40-bulb LED flashlight lasts up to 24 hours if fully charged. Install LED lamps throughout your home; you turn on these LED lamps during a blackout. Since modern LED lights are very bright, your home will be well-illuminated throughout the outage.

Avoid opening your refrigerator if you don't have to get something inside. You need to maintain the coolness inside your fridge for as long as possible to keep the contents fresh and bacteria-free.

Electric generators should never be kept and operated inside the house. If you want a generator, place it outside, in a protected spot, away from moisture, children, and pets, and operate it there. Your home will be safe if something goes wrong or the generator suddenly catches fire.

Electrical generators work best if you connect the electrical equipment you need to use directly to the various outlets in the generator. Do not directly hook your home's main power line to the generator because this might overload it. An overloaded generator will stall or, worse, overheat and possibly catch fire.

Use battery-operated radios and television sets to listen to local news to get updates.

Emergency services (911) respond to life-threatening situations at any time of the day. Please do not call them to ask how long the blackout will last.

They might know (or know who to call), but it is not their job to relay such information. If there is a rolling blackout and you want to know when it will be over, call the utility company instead.

If it becomes freezing because of no heat, add additional layers of clothing to keep warm. Do not use your oven as an 'instant furnace." It is also a bad idea to burn charcoal inside the house so that you can cook if you are using electric stoves and the like. Suppose you want to use charcoal, grill, or cook outside food.

Pets can become dehydrated if it gets too hot or cold inside your home. Remember to give them fresh water to drink.

SAFETY DURING A HAZARDOUS MATERIALS INCIDENT

It's a fact of life – modern society has become entirely dependent on using different chemical compounds to accomplish specific goals, such as creating higher-yielding crops, improving the quality of the water that runs through our faucets, and so on.

There is nothing wrong with the proper use of chemicals. Indeed, the convenient and comfortable life we now enjoy partly results from using different industrial compounds and chemical materials.

However, there are times when the chemicals that help society move along endanger whole communities.

A hazardous materials incident manifests when vast amounts of chemicals are mishandled or accidentally released into the environment.

That is considered a disaster not only for the environment but also for people. Industrial chemicals, such as mercury (used to fabricate items like light bulbs), can cause serious health problems.

If such chemicals were handled and stored correctly, there would be no threat to the public. But what should you do if an HMI does manifest? The following section deals with this pressing question.

HMI SAFETY GUIDELINES

Local authorities treat HMIs very seriously because if the HM is toxic to people, far-reaching health consequences may threaten the public. The authorities will most likely advise the community to do one or several things during an HMI.

Local authorities will ask people to evacuate their homes.

If you are advised to evacuate, do so immediately. Don't wait three or ten hours before abandoning your home because you must pack stuff before leaving. That puts your and everyone else's lives in your hands. If local authorities ask families to leave their homes, that means there is an immediate health risk due to the HMI. Evacuation routes will be set up by the local authorities. Have a radio or portable television to monitor announcements from the authorities and local emergency personnel. You can go to the designated evacuation shelters or arrange temporary lodging elsewhere during evacuations. It's up to you – people won't force you to drive to emergency evacuation shelters. Just make sure that your choice of temporary accommodation is as far away as possible from the site of the HMI. If your neighbors seem unaware of what's happening, devote a few minutes to tell them what's happening so they can make the necessary preparations.

If there is an HMI and you are still far from home.

If you are very near the site of the HMI, drive or walk

somewhere upwind. Air can carry toxic chemicals far and wide, so an upwind area is necessary to keep yourself safe. Half a mile is a reasonable distance from an HMI site. If you can go farther, do it. If you are in an area where you see solid particles and chemical mists all around you, do not touch them, and minimize inhalation! Cover your face as much as possible with cloth, and keep walking. It is foolhardy to inspect any chemicals lying on the ground - don't even think of touching the stuff because we don't know what it is (unless the authorities have already announced what exactly has happened). If you see people who are injured by chemicals, do not try to go near them! It's one thing to call 911 to ask for help, but it's an entirely different proposition when you come near someone to tend to their wounds. That's too much risk for you; let emergency personnel respond. The best thing that you can contribute to the situation is a call to 911. That is enough help.

An HMI is announced while you are driving home from/ to work.

Unless you are already very far from the site of the HMI (say ½ mile at least), park your vehicle somewhere upstream and wait for further announcements. It might be dangerous to drive further because the chemicals may have already spread through the air. During this time, it is wise to turn off the air-conditioning in your car because it requires using the car's vents. Vents can let in chemicals lingering in the air. All doors and windows must be shut, too. Put up with the heat – it is well worth the wait. Also, turn off the engine to conserve gas. You never know how much traveling you will do now that an HMI is in progress.

Local authorities advise everyone to stay home and only venture outside once further announcements are made.

Kids and pets should come inside; no exceptions. Pets are equally at risk during HMIs. If a person can suffocate or suffer from nervous system damage, so can animals like cats and dogs. Doors, windows, and other vents should be locked tightly. Your home's air-conditioning and ventilation systems should be turned off temporarily until authorities say the danger has passed. This guideline is because air from the outside can quickly get inside if the ventilation system is still on. You do not want that to happen during an HMI.

BIOLOGICAL WARFARE

Terrorist organizations may use biological agents, such as anthrax, to strike fear among the population. While the federal government does its best to prevent such attacks, it is still possible that terrorist groups can strike anywhere in the country.

As citizens, we must protect ourselves from such threats because, in the end, our knowledge of these threats is what will save us from possible illness or death.

Biological warfare involves the use of microorganisms and toxic chemicals to harm people, animals, and crops.

History has taught us how people can become creative with biological agents. Biological agents spread through the air, water, and even food. Toxic agents can also be delivered through aerosol cans.

SAFETY GUIDELINES DURING A BIOLOGICAL ATTACK

Monitor the news for any updates regarding the possible biological attack. Local and national authorities usually take their time formulating updates for the public, so don't expect to get all the information you need in just one news update.

The authorities will provide updates every hour regarding the situation, so it is best to leave the radio or TV on to receive them as they are broadcast.

If you find a suspicious material or substance nearby, don't try to inspect it visually or touch it. Get away from it quickly. The longer you stay in the vicinity, the higher the toxin/bacteria exposure risk.

If you're outdoors during a possible biological attack, you need to protect your eyes, nose, mouth, and ears, as these orifices are targets for toxins and other rogue biological agents. Exposed skin, such as your hands, legs, and arms, should be covered, too, at the very least, by a thin piece of cloth.

What should you do if you have already been exposed? All your clothes and stuff you have been carrying should be disposed of appropriately.

Yes, you have to throw away clothing and even your bag. Local authorities will probably release a bulletin outlining the proper method of disposing of such items after a possible/

actual biological attack.

When you come home after exposure, you should first take a long bath. Scrub yourself well with soap, and put on fresh, clean clothes.

Most biological agents die when they come into contact with sunlight, water, etc. That's why it is vital to take a bath quickly to rid your skin of any lingering toxins or microorganisms that may cause harm later on.

Do not expose others to the same risk if you have been exposed severely. Contact emergency personnel and inform them what happened. You may be asked to quarantine until emergency personnel arrive to help decontaminate and treat you.

A biological attack may or may not produce illness and health hazards. It's good to be suspicious if you or someone else in the family gets sick all of a sudden after a possible biological attack. But this doesn't mean a biological attack causes every symptom you feel. Don't run to the emergency room whenever you think something odd (i.e., you have a sudden cold).

Local authorities will post a list of symptoms related to identified biological agents. If you find some symptoms have manifested, contact emergency personnel immediately.

TERRORIST ATTACKS & EXPLOSIVES

Many terrorist bombings have marred the history of the World. The dire memory of them all has left scars on the collective psyche of humanity everywhere. That is why we should also be prepared to protect ourselves in the event of a terrorist bombing.

Explosives Facts.

The technology of bomb-making has become highly advanced in the past few decades. Explosives that pack a massive payload during detonation can be carried in small suitcases or strapped on by terrorist members.

Explosives are lightweight and often innocuous-looking; that is what makes these explosives twice as deadly because most folks won't even know that there is a bomb in a public place until the blast occurs.

Bombs can be transported by small cars, large trucks (i.e., Oklahoma City bombing), and individuals. Explosives can even be strapped on a human body, along with the wiring.

Bombs can be left in public places and detonated wirelessly using a remote bomb trigger. Bombs can also be placed in public utility vehicles, such as buses and trains, to cause the most harm to public infrastructure (i.e., train tracks) and people.

Bomb attacks can happen anywhere and anytime; terrorists tend to move when the public is at ease and unsuspecting.

HANDLING A BOMB THREAT

Bomb threats can be real or just pranks. We all hope that they are pranks because pranks can be rendered harmless by their intended recipients.

But if you receive a telephone call from someone aware of a bomb placed in your building or a building nearby, you need to get as much information as possible from the person on the other end of the line. You can ask the following questions.

When is the bomb going to be detonated?

What is the location of the explosive device?

What does the explosive device look like?

What kind of explosive device has been placed in the building?

What would trigger the explosion of the bomb?

Is the caller the person responsible for placing the explosive device?

There is no assurance that the caller will be cooperative and answer all these questions, but it's good to try; who knows, the person might answer some questions and give you vital information that will aid the authorities later on.

Before saying goodbye, write down everything you hear in a notebook or paper. Right after receiving the bomb threat, call 911 and relay the information you collected over the phone. Spare no detail.

Do not be afraid to relay the information to the authorities. It is also a good idea to call someone at the target building to inform them of what you have just learned. Time is pure gold when there is a bomb threat; one never knows when the bomber will detonate the explosive device.

CHARACTERISTICS OF SUSPICIOUS AND POTENTIALLY DEADLY PACKAGES

Over the years, professional postal inspectors and local authorities have amassed a list of features that make a package or parcel suspicious.

Suspicious parcels may or may not contain explosives, and there's a 50/50 chance, so you should contact the authorities immediately if you find a suspicious package.

Do not open or approach suspicious parcels or packages! The following are some characteristics of packages that should arouse your suspicion.

You receive a package from someone you do not know.

The package itself does not have a return address.

Strange notes are written on the package, such as "Do Not Xray." Such signage is usually meant to prevent postal inspectors from discovering what is inside.

The package smells strange.

The package has protruding metal wires.

The postmark on the package does not match the return address that is also written on the box.

The package has an odd weight.

The package has an odd shape.

The package has been marked with a threatening message.

You feel the package's contents have been wrapped in

excessive bubble wrap, paper, or strings.

The message on the package has strange misspellings.

The package has been addressed to someone in your home, company, or business who left long ago.

Addresses present on the package have been handwritten (and poorly, at that).

SURVIVING A BLAST

If there is a bomb blast, think and act fast to keep yourself safe until you can relocate yourself as far away as possible from the blast site. Here are some additional guidelines.

If debris falls from the ceiling, find a suitable cover, such as a sturdy table, and get underneath. Cover your face and your head to protect yourself from flying debris.

Explosions are intended to harm the most significant number of people and cause structural damage. Part of the building where the explosion occurred may be weakened significantly after the blast. You must leave the building as quickly and safely as possible because there might be additional blasts.

If you are on a building's top floor, you should use the stairs, not the elevators, to go down. Stairs are safer; elevators may malfunction or have been rigged.

Observe your surroundings. Is there a fire starting somewhere close to you?

Once you are out of a bombed building, get as far away as possible from the site. Stay away from windows and doors, as these will undoubtedly shatter or explode if a fire occurs.

If you find yourself trapped by fallen debris, use your cell phone or a small flashlight to signal to rescuers. Avoid unnecessary movement, and don't breathe in excessive dust.

EMERGENCY KIT

The following are supplies and equipment that should be assembled beforehand. This emergency kit can be used in any disaster scenario.

Medications, glasses or contact lenses, milk formulas, diapers, food, and water for your pets.

Vital documents, such as birth certificates and bank-related documents.

Cash. Credit Cards. Traveler's checks. Spare change.

First-aid manual. A thick blanket for each person in the family. A sleeping bag for each person in the family.

Comfortable and protective clothing for yourself and your family. Bleach. Fire extinguisher (ABC type). Matches. Personal care items.

Paper plates, disposable spoons, forks, and paper towels.

Notebook or paper. Pen. Items that can be used by children to entertain themselves.

A gallon of fresh water for each member of the family.

Three days supply of food Battery-operated TV. Battery-operated radio. Extra batteries. Flashlight. Whistle. First-aid kit.

There should be a dust mask for each family member, garbage bags, pliers, a can opener, maps, and spare mobile phones with fully charged batteries.

SUMMING UP

What Are the Two Kinds of Floods?

Floods can happen anytime and anywhere, so it's best to be prepared to deal with one no matter where you reside in the country. There are two general classes of floods.

The first kind is regular flooding, often after a torrential downpour. You have time to prepare for this flooding, and you can seek higher ground if necessary. The second type of flood is called a flash flood.

Flash floods carry not only large amounts of water but also a myriad of debris from other places. We're talking about tree branches, raw sewage (in some cases), and lots of mud. Flash floods are especially deadly when they come down on homes that have been constructed at the foot of a mountain or even the foot of a small hill.

It can come at any time, so if there's a storm and you live in a place where flash floods have occurred before, someone in your household must monitor the situation around the clock. Most fatalities associated with flash floods arise from people caught sleeping in torrential water and mud.

Monitoring a dire weather situation is as simple as staying tuned to the local news channel so you can receive hourly bulletins. You can also watch the weather online to see if the power hasn't been knocked out or if the area has no rolling blackouts due to inclement weather.

What Causes Flooding?

Heavy rain or storms are the common causes of flooding. In some situations, a powerful hurricane can bring a deadly storm surge that can quickly submerge whole communities.

The problem with floods is that they carry water and small and large particles of debris from different places. If the flood occurs in a highly populated area, the chances of raw sewage mixing with floodwater increase significantly. It's one thing to navigate through six inches of water, but what if you have to walk through floodwater with raw sewage and other unsanitary things?

Another potential cause of the flooding is melted snow and ice. Spring flooding is relatively frequent in areas with natural bodies of water. When the ice melts due to the increasingly warm environment, rivers, streams, and ponds overflow. You might be wondering: shouldn't the ground absorb all that water?

Unfortunately, the ground is still mostly frozen during early spring, so it won't be able to absorb the extra water. Water has to go somewhere, so once a stream or spring overflows, the excess water will have to flow away from the main body of water. Another common cause of flooding is a problem with the dam. Dam operators may have to release water when a dam becomes jammed by ice or is at risk of overflowing due to excess rainfall. Excess water can flood nearby communities because dams release several gallons of water per minute.

Drive Safely Through a Flooded Area

During heavy downpours, you may have to drive through flooded roads and areas on your way home. If the water rises and you do not know what's happening at home, you will want to drive back to check on your family.

If you are about to drive through a flooded area, first check the height of the floodwater. You can drive through it without stalling if it is under six inches.

Most cars will stall when the exhaust pipe is filled with water. If the floodwater is over six inches tall, your car will stall unless you have a big SUV or an all-terrain, four-wheel drive with large wheels. If the floodwater is 12 inches in height or more, your car may float when you attempt to drive through the flood, so don't try it.

Park where the flood will not reach you, and then try to think of other ways to communicate with your family. Remember: you won't be able to help others if you're stranded on a flooded road. If your car stalls, you will have to take care of it yourself and your car because you won't be able to operate it anymore.

Are You Ready for an Earthquake?

Earthquakes are one of Mother Nature's most destructive natural phenomena. Like floods, they can rock and devastate whole communities (or cities) in the blink of an eye. Earthquakes occur when massive sheets of hard rock underneath the earth's surface shift and collide.

This titanic movement on the planet's surface can generate large amounts of seismic energy. Energy doesn't just disappear when it is produced; it is transmitted, and there has to be some outlet for it. Unfortunately, when seismic energy is created, we feel its presence by the violent shaking of the ground.

If the earth were uninhabited, earthquakes would be minor disturbances on the planet's crust. However, since the World is inhabited by billions of people, earthquakes can be a real problem because, during an earthquake, large buildings, roads, and bridges tend to crack or collapse.

While it is true that earthquakes can become deadly, you don't have to worry too much if you are adept at disaster preparedness. Take steps to ensure you survive even the worst earthquakes.

For example, people run for cover during an earthquake, thinking the outdoors is the best place to seek refuge. If you are indoors, stay indoors. First, you should find a sturdy cover so falling debris won't hit you. A large table is an excellent cover. If you cannot find a good cover, find a safe corner of the room and cover your head with your arms instead.

Keep Yourself Safe During an Earthquake

Not all earthquakes are deadly or destructive. Indeed, seismologists record dozens of micro earthquakes every single day. The general populace never feels these mini-quakes because they generate too little seismic energy. On the other hand, some earthquakes can cause destruction. These earthquakes have a magnitude of six to ten on the Richter scale. The higher the magnitude of a shock, the more destructive it can become.

An earthquake of nine can cause destruction hundreds of miles from the quake's epicenter. Expect the ground to move continuously if you face a magnitude five (or higher) earthquake.

Don't try to save stuff from falling because all of the items in your home that have been elevated will most likely fall off their shelves. Instead, find a safe room (like the bedroom) with no hanging light fixtures or heavy, elevated items. You should also avoid windows and doors with glass in them.

Glass can easily break and shatter during earthquakes because of the erratic ground movement. While this doesn't always happen, it is best to assume that it can happen so there won't be any earthquake-related accidents.

If you want to keep your appliances safe from earthquakes, you can either strap them to the wall or permanently bolt them to the floor. That takes some time and effort, but it is well worth it. Also, make it a habit to place heavy items near the floor and not on top of shelves so you won't have to dodge heavy "missiles" during a strong earthquake.

Don't Let an Earthquake Endanger Your Life

We've previously discussed the preliminary steps you can take in an earthquake. This lesson will discuss further steps to keep you safe in a strong quake.

If the earthquake strikes while you are still in the bedroom, don't leave your bedroom. Instead, go back to bed and find the biggest pillow so you have something to cover your head. Stay on the bed until the earthquake passes unless you have a hanging light fixture that might fall on you. If there is a light fixture on the ceiling above your bed, go to a corner of your bedroom that is as far away from the light fixture and glass windows. Crouch in that corner and protect your head with your arms or a pillow.

If you are in a building, pass through doorways quickly. Stay away from doors because unless a doorway or gate has been specifically designed to handle large loads and stresses, it can collapse or crumple at any time. You don't want to get hit by a collapsing doorframe.

Do not use the elevators if you need to descend from the top of a building. Take the stairs because they are always safer. It doesn't matter if it takes a few more minutes to go down on foot. Elevators are dangerous during earthquakes because the cables may snap, and you might end up hurtling several meters per second toward the ground floor.

Are You Prepared for a Heat Wave?

Excessive heat, or a heat wave, occurs when the temperature in a given area is 100 to 110 degrees Fahrenheit (37 to 43 Celsius). This temperature can cause heat exhaustion, cramps, and even heat stroke. People who work outdoors should take extra precautions when there is a heat wave because the body can succumb to excessive heat without warning. You should monitor changes in the weather by tuning in to your local news channel.

That will allow you to receive bulletins from the authorities, who will tell you what to do during the heat wave (if experts advise special precautions). When an excessive heat warning is broadcasted, a heat wave is coming within one to three days.

It's difficult to pinpoint the exact hour of a heat wave because factors that affect the weather change regularly, and meteorologists can only do so much with their monitoring equipment. During a heat wave, temperatures rise to 43 degrees Celsius (or 109 degrees Fahrenheit, which is way above the average body temperature).

This kind of temperature can easily cause illness and exhaustion in children, so ensure your kids aren't exposed to this heat during the heat wave. Adults should also take necessary precautions, such as staying indoors and getting plenty of fluids.

Safety Guidelines During Periods of Excessive Heat

Disaster preparedness is all about getting the correct information to know what to do during a disaster or emergency. If you are prepared for a disaster, you know how to keep yourself safe and safeguard the health and lives of those around you. That is a pressing need, especially if you have children at home. Children will entirely depend on your knowledge and actions during an emergency; they have no one else to rely on but you. Let's discuss a few essential safety guidelines that should always be remembered during periods of excessive heat.

Children should never be left in the car for prolonged periods, even if the air conditioning is on. The heat from the immediate environment can quickly get into the vehicle, and this additional heat can cause heat exhaustion or muscle cramps.

Heat waves are often accompanied by excessive humidity. Proper air conditioning at home is essential to be comfortable throughout the heat wave. Heat waves can last for days sometimes; you want to avoid excessive heat that long.

If you must go out during a heat wave, choose wide-open

locations with adequate ventilation. Going to the mall is a good idea, too, because it's air-conditioned and spacious. Most public libraries are excellent, too.

How Do You Know If a Landslide Is Coming?

Landslides typically occur in areas with steep slopes and bodies of water. Storms and heavy downpours can cause landslides. Sometimes, they happen because of prolonged periods of erosion. If your home is standing on a steep slope or has been built at the bottom of a valley or mountain, you may experience a landslide if sufficient factors come into play. You should be aware of several warning signs.

Geographical landscapes are always in a state of change. However, if there is an accelerated change in your environment, erosion may occur faster, too. If the slope of the land suddenly changes for no reason, a landslide might occur.

If your home is built on a steep slope, jammed doors and windows indicate that the soil underneath your house is changing. If the ground shifts, soil in other parts of the area may also be shifting. Moving earth can mean an imminent landslide. It might not happen within twenty-four hours, but it may happen soon.

Your home's foundation is the only part directly interacting with the ground soil. If cracks suddenly emerge in your foundation, that may mean that the soil underneath your house is being eroded or is shifting. That is a bad sign because if the ground underneath your home is moving, your home may change along with it.

Beware of the Dangers of Wildfires

Wildfires, or firestorms, are regular occurrences in parts of the United States where the land is generally dry and temperatures are consistently high. Fires can destroy hundreds upon hundreds of acres of land, and, as experience has already taught us, it's not easy to contain a wildfire because you are dealing not only with an almost inexhaustible amount of fuel or combustible materials but several other factors (like wind) that help make fires broader and more aggressive.

Irresponsible burning and accidents often cause wildfires in prairies and grasslands. Sometimes, even forests burn down in a fire, especially if there are few hardwood trees in the area. If you live somewhere near meadows, be aware that wildfires can occur instantaneously, even without someone lighting a match or a campfire. In a fire, you should first call emergency services to inform them of a wildfire in your area.

The faster someone can call emergency services, the quicker the firemen arrive to put out the fire. That applies especially to wildfires that are incredibly close to residential areas because once a few houses catch fire, it is common for the fire to spread to other homes if no fire-stopping measures are implemented.

If a wildfire is nearby, close all windows and doors, but don't lock them if firefighters have to enter your home later. Have a long garden hose ready to douse any materials that may have caught fire. Leaving your home and arranging temporary lodging elsewhere is best if the fire finally reaches your house.

APPENDIX

What is the Cause of a Heat Wave?

No single factor produces extreme heat, or heat waves, in any location in the world. A heat wave emerges if there is a sudden and often prolonged increase in the average temperature of any given area compared to its average temperature throughout the years.

Since heat causes water to evaporate rapidly from the Earth, excessive heat is also frequently accompanied by high humidity. High humidity can also increase the impact of a heat wave as it rolls across a town or city.

In the United States, temperatures between 40 and 44 degrees Celsius are considered markers of a heat wave. If your local news channel announces that there will be excessive heat soon, that means the heat wave will manifest in one to three days.

When there is an incoming heat wave, limiting your exposure to direct sunlight is essential. If you have to work under the sun for long periods, it is best to be accompanied by someone in case something happens to you.

Remember: the longer a person remains exposed to the sun during excessive heat or a heat wave, the higher the chances of suffering heat exhaustion, heat stroke, muscle cramps, etc.

There are so many problems medical problems associated with excessive heat that you should protect yourself nicely.

Guidelines for Excessive Heat

You must keep your whole family safe during a heat wave. Here are some steps to ensure everyone is healthy and happy throughout the heat wave.

1. If you live in a warm region of the country and have air conditioning installed, ensure that the insulation around the air conditioning unit and the insulation around the house is in good condition. Poor insulation can cause the temperatures inside the home to rise, placing additional strain on your air conditioning unit.

2. Weather-stripping entrances and exits can also help keep the heat out.

3. Windows facing the sun from morning until late afternoon should be covered with heavy material, such as drapes, to keep out the sun's rays. The sun's rays can automatically increase your home's temperature, so it is best to block them with drapes.

4. Storm windows, on the other hand, should be kept open to ensure proper air circulation throughout the home.

5. You must keep updated with the latest news about the heat wave, so keep listening to the radio and watching your local news channel. Alternatively, you can download a reliable weather app on mobile to check (hourly) any temperature changes.

6. Taking quick and frequent showers throughout the day can help regulate body temperature and relieve heat exhaustion. Do this if you must go out during a heat wave for errands. If you want to go out during the excessive heat (even if you don't have to), go to air-conditioning structures like the mall or the city library.

Calamity Preparedness Information

Calamity can strike at any time. If you want to keep yourself and those around you safe when it suddenly strikes, you need to make sure that you have all of the necessary information you will need to survive the disaster in the first place.

There are generally two types of disasters: natural and human-made.

Natural disasters include hurricanes, typhoons, floods, and volcanic eruptions. Human-made disasters, on the other hand, can consist of biological attacks, hazardous materials incidents, and even terrorist attacks. In an emergency, keeping yourself and your family safe is possible.

General guidelines for disaster preparedness.

1. Create an emergency supplies kit for the entire family. Supplies included in this kit consist of complete changes of clothes for each member of the family. Each family member needs at least one gallon of water. Flashlights or rechargeable LED lamps. Food supplies that won't spoil quickly, even without refrigeration. Important personal documents, such as bank account records and birth certificates. Extra cash (not credit cards), sleeping bags, blankets, mattresses, pillows, and any prescription medication you or any other family member may need.

2. In a disaster, you must be aware of any public announcements or bulletins from the local authorities. By local authorities, we refer specifically to emergency services personnel, such as the police and the fire brigade.

These departments may periodically send out bulletins to inform the public of any changes in the situation. Local agencies often transmit bulletins over the radio, television, and Internet.

3. If you must drive to a safe location during a disaster, ensure that the roads and other areas you will be passing through are safe before proceeding. Driving through flooded areas is generally not a good idea, but if you have to do it, try to measure just how deep the flood is.

If the flood is less than six inches tall, you can drive through it and survive. But if the wave is more than six inches in height, there is a good chance that your car will stall.

If the water is over six inches tall, it has been known to stall and even carry away sports utility vehicles. Do not underestimate the power of muddy water; you can get hurt doing it.

4. In case of a human-made disaster (such as a biological attack or a hazardous materials incident), staying at an up-wind location is best.

Chemical and biological agents can travel through the air, so it is best to steer clear of the affected area until the authorities have announced that the emergency is over. People can resume normal activities without fearing contamination or disease.

If you think you have come into contact with hazardous waste or a biological agent, go to a hospital's emergency unit and have yourself checked out. That is the only way to ensure you are safe and won't need any special procedures after exposure.

What are the Effects of Landslides?

Landslides can quickly destroy personal property, like houses and vehicles, and significantly change an area's landscape. They also threaten agriculture, livestock, and local businesses because once a steady debris flow emerges, there is no way to block its advance into residential, commercial, or even agricultural areas. Flash floods often bring large amounts of mud and debris, so be prepared for a landslide if there is a flash flood in your area. Safety guidelines.

1. Be aware of the common signs of an impending landslide: new cracks in your home's foundation, sudden jamming of different windows and doors, changes in your property's global landscape, sinking land, the appearance of water in places where water has never flowed before, and so on. Any unexpected change in the landscape may signal that the area is changing and

shifting.

2. As mentioned earlier, flooding can trigger a massive landslide or debris flow. If you know that an incoming storm is strong enough to blow down houses, there is no point in sleeping through the storm. You might become the victim of a sudden landslide if you don't monitor the situation.

Monitoring your surroundings for signs of a landslide is essential if you have small children and pets to take care of. You won't be able to organize a quick and safe evacuation if you are startled awake in the middle of the night only to discover that the landslide has already breached your doors and windows.

3. If you are in the middle of an avalanche, move away from the debris flow path as soon as possible. Refrain from wasting time trying to gather clothes and other non-essential items.

Make a quick and safe escape, and keep running (or driving) until you are as far away as possible from the strongest point of the debris flow. You can make all the repairs you want later on in your house, but when faced with an actual landslide, your priority is to get away from the mudflow as quickly as possible.

4. If you live in the country or near valleys and mountains, the safest areas are the ones that are higher than where you live right now. Stay away from areas lower than your property because these places will likely become catch basins for the debris flow. Landslides are composed of mud and lots and lots of water.

This water makes the debris flow viscous, making it twice as dangerous in the grand scheme because it can travel much faster than just falling rocks or uprooted trees.

5. It is common for massive landslides to generate smaller landslides (the same way earthquakes produce aftershocks), so don't go back to your home immediately after an avalanche. Wait for the authorities to declare the entire area safe before returning to your house. Until such time, stay at a designated shelter or stay in a hotel. Your home can wait.

The Basics of Flood Survival

Flooding is a natural disaster that has touched nearly every country or locale. It has always been a problem, and it will not go away, even with the advent of global warming, because the hydrological cycle will still exist; the environment will always recycle water through rain and storms.

Since we can't do anything about the natural phenomena that regularly cause flooding, we can only be prepared for flooding when it occurs.

There are two general types of floods. The first type is the regular flood, which occurs after long periods of rain. The water level in the immediate land area steadily rises until the water has to flow where the land's slope is lower.

Then we have flash floods. Flash floods are far more sinister than regular waves because they can submerge a whole neighborhood in minutes without warning.

That is one of the reasons why you should stay awake in the advent of a massive storm. A flash flood can come from anywhere, and even if you are far away from their usual sites, water can still reach you if sufficient water (and debris) comes in from a higher area.

Safety During a Flood

Floods can destroy property and take lives just as quickly, so being in a flood-prone area is no laughing matter. If you have just moved to a new city or neighborhood, asking your neighbors if the area has experienced any recent flooding might be a good idea.

If it has experienced flooding before, even if the flood took place five years ago, then it is likely that a big storm can cause a surge in the area again. It doesn't matter if the last flood was ages ago; the mere fact that the region has been flooded before means the geographical topography of the area is susceptible to flooding.

And, unless extremely large counter-measures have already been taken to ensure that the landscape does not encourage flash floods and regular floods, it is still not safe to assume that flooding in your neighborhood is not possible.

If you live in a house with a second or third floor, move essential items to the upper floors during a storm so that these items will be safe even if it does flood.

Also, avoid driving through flooded areas because your vehicle might stall, and you could get stuck in the middle of nowhere during a flood. Beware of six to twelve inches of water, enough to stall and float a one-ton vehicle.

Electricity and water must be turned off during a flood to minimize problems. The wave will eventually subside, and you can turn on these utilities after a few hours.

Hospital Disaster Plans: Primer

City and county hospitals are usually the first places people flock to in disasters and emergencies. Each hospital must have an effective plan that can be implemented quickly in case a full-scale disaster suddenly manifests.

1. The purpose of a hospital disaster plan is to respond promptly to disaster situations, both arising from within the hospital and accidents arising externally. A hospital disaster plan must be implemented immediately if a disaster threatens a hospital staff, doctors, nurses, or patients.

2. During a disaster, it is imperative that each hospital staff member has an assigned responsibility or task during the emergency.

3. It is ideal if the team reviews the standard operating guidelines of the hospital in question.

4. The following disasters can affect a hospital: HMI (hazardous materials incidents), large fires, earthquakes, landslides, flash floods, etc. Emergencies that can affect the community can also affect a nearby hospital; a neighboring disaster becomes a hospital disaster if the safety of the

personnel and patients are put at risk.

5. The hospital shall establish a central control center where all vital communications will be passed through the proper channels.

6. Visitors shall be given access to a separate control center. This control center will be the general space where relatives and friends of patients can wait for any critical notifications if they have any patients in the hospital.

7. The hospital shall ensure that anyone who needs to make or receive a call from that location has access to a working telephone line.

8. Any extra required supplies shall be acquired through delivery and the service of runners.

9. In a large-scale disaster, the hospital may offer free rooms or areas as a public control center for reporters and the media.

The hospital must also set up a system of transmitting information through TV and radio in case public announcements and warnings have to be communicated to the public.

10. In case of large-scale disasters, the hospital administration must communicate with the local authorities to confirm the areas affected and the scale of the accident.

The hospital must also work closely with the police and all other emergency personnel so that any victims of the current disaster can be quickly brought into the hospital. The hospital will be code orange throughout the accident, and staff must be prepared to accept large numbers of patients at any time.

11. All departments must report to the command center in preparation for any required actions during the disaster.

12. All nursing aids must be present and able to provide first aid measures to patients who need it. During a catastrophe, no hospital staff shall leave a patient's side unless the patient has been formally signed off. Disaster numbers should be assigned to each patient (even if the patient has been cleared as 'dead on arrival').

What are Landslides?

Landslides, or debris falls, are the continuous movement of mud and debris from a higher location down to a land area with a lower slope. Landslides can take place after a light rain, or they can take place even if there is no rainfall.

A landslide can carry water, mud, uprooted trees, garbage, and, sometimes, raw sewage. The composition of an avalanche, or debris flow, depends on where it originated. If the debris flows from a mountain, it can only carry water, rocks, mud, and maybe some trees.

However, if the debris flow is coming in from an urban area, then there may be some raw sewage that may have been collected along the way. Landslides are extremely dangerous regardless of their composition because they can carry away whole vehicles and houses with weak foundations.

Safety Tips

If you live in an area with frequent landslides, you must protect yourself and your property. If your home is built on a steep slope or at the very bottom of a hill or mountain, then you must have your house checked by a professional inspector every six months to see if it is holding up well to the terrain on which it was built.

Any new cracks in your home's foundation should be considered suspicious. Only earthquakes can cause multiple cracks in a house's foundation. Soft and shifting soil is another indicator of an impending landslide.

If the land around your house feels softer than usual, and there hasn't been any rain, it is possible that the soil in other parts of the area has already shifted, and a landslide is imminent. We must remember that avalanches don't give out warning signals, and one can happen immediately if the correct number of factors come into play.

During a landslide, your priority is to get out of the debris flow path. If you think the landslide will destroy your house, it probably will, but it won't matter if you and your family are safe. You can do little to reduce the onslaught of an incoming landslide, so don't stay home to try to reduce its impact.

It only won't work. If you get caught in the path of a landslide and you cannot move, seek cover, curl yourself tightly into the form of a ball, and stay put. If you can make a run for it, do not go downhill; go uphill instead, where the debris flow will be less intense.

Remember: mud and water like to go down because of the pull of gravity. The safest places are elevated ones. If you have a car and can drive away, don't steer toward the debris flow; drive away from it. So, if the landslide is heading south, drive up north.

THE END

ABOUT THE AUTHOR

Andrea Scarsi is a master of meditation who defines himself as a mystic, metaphysician, author, musician, and holistic coach when he uses his works to share a dimension of being, lifestyle, and knowledge founded on communion with the absolute.

Born in Venice, Italy, in 1955, he began practicing yoga and spiritism and experimenting with telepathy at fifteen. Following a near-death experience, he contacted alien and transdimensional entities at eighteen. At twenty-four, on his first trip to India, he found himself a vegetarian and in the world of meditation led by India and the Spiritual Master Osho. He received Swami Prem Sandesh as a new name, which he wears in specific environments.

He has often traveled, especially to India, residing for long periods in Nepal, the Philippines, Brazil, and Buddhist Southeast Asia: Japan, Thailand, Sri Lanka, Hong Kong, Laos, China, and Tibet. He has explored local places and cultures, met people, and participated in ritual and religious practices.

Over time, he delved into various meditative techniques for awakening consciousness, energy rebalancing, and personal evolution, which he practices and teaches. He studied philosophy and earned a Doctorate in Metaphysical Science and various diplomas, such as Holistic Life Coach, Reiki Grand Master, Master of Crystals, Shamanism, Meditation and Massage, and Wellness Coach. He's also into cellular nutrition and Network Marketing.

In 1991, he married Krisana, and they now live in Venice, Italy. Reach him at andrea.scarsi@yahoo.com and https://www.youtube.com/@ScarsiAndrea.

BOOKS BY ANDREA SCARSI

About Osho
Answers For The Soul
Blessings!
Dead Man Walking
Extraterrestrial Channeling
Happy To Be Happy
Holistic Massage
Holistic Wellness
Home Sweet Home Staging
How I Restore My Brain Abilities
How To Ask A Woman Out
Imagine
Indigo Crystal Rainbow and Diamond
Journey To The Underworld
Make Your Own Vineyard
O Iguana! My Iguana!
Orchids Beauty Meditation
Overweight? No Problem!
Pearls of Wisdom
Reiki First Degree Manual
Reiki Second Degree Manual
Reiki Third Degree Manual
Romance Ain't Love Pollution
Seeds Of Enlightenment
Stop Dreaming
Swimming in The Ganges
Tarot Reading Essentials
The Art of Change
The Art of Persuasion
The Art of Worrying
The Depths Of Stillness And The Art Of Dissolving
The Foolproof Way to Fail at Online Trading
The Magic Of Money

The Master And The Assassin
The Secret Of Meditation
The Secret Of Metaphysical Science
The Silence of The Absolute
Vegetarian Cuisine
Walking The Dogs
Zen The Sense Of Nonsense

MANTRAS BY SANDESH (ANDREA SCARSI)

Mantras Mahamantras
The Mantra Experiment
The Mantra Way
Om Namo Supernova
Amavasya
Lingamananda

A mantra is a Verbal Being acting as a bridge between the human and the divine. It carries our prayer, thankfulness, and gratitude. It is an entity in its own right, and when we recite or sing it to communicate with the superior dimension, in addition to words and sound, we also employ intention, energy, devotion, and focus. All this raises us immediately. It increases our emotional state and makes us touch God.

A mantra is an introspective event turning to the multiple aspects of the One by evoking its symbolic names: Shiva, Brahma, Vishnu, Ganesha, Laxmi, Saraswati, Gurudev, Shanti; names representing the infinite manifestation of the cosmic cycle. They are magic formulas for amending the universal present, resolving the apparent fragmentation, and recreating the union of consciousness with what is.

A mantra is to be recited and sung without interruption, to convey the intact message, and breathing comes between recitations. Let's get lost in the mantra, and let the vehicle, the human, and the divine become one. That's the power of mantra. We recite it and go deeper, until melting what we were before, our intention, recitation, sound, and collective energy, and manifesting unity once again, the yoga of consciousness, the absolute presence, whose supreme name is Om.

BOOKS BY ANDREA SCARSI IN ITALIAN

21 Giorni
A Proposito di Osho
Basta Sognare
Benedizioni!
Benessere Olistico
Benvenuti ad Atlantide
Breve Storia Dei Sogni
Canalizzazioni Extraterrestri
Casa Dolce Casa Vendesi
Come Ripristino Le Capacità Del Mio Cervello
Dhyana Yoga
Dispense Reiki Primo Livello
Dispense Reiki Secondo Livello
Dispense Reiki Terzo Livello Master
Felici Di Essere Felici
Guarire il Sé Ombra
Il Lato Positronico
Il Maestro e l'Assassino
Il Modo Infallibile Per Fallire Nel Trading Online
Il Romanticismo Non è Inquinamento Emotivo
Il Segreto della Meditazione
Il Segreto della Scienza Metafisica
Il Silenzio dell'Assoluto
Immagina
Indaco Cristallo Arcobaleno e Diamante
La Cucina Vegetariana
L'Arte della Persuasione
L'Arte della Preoccupazione
L'Arte di Cambiare
L'Arte di Invitare una Donna
Le Acque sacre del Gange
Le Compatibilità Zodiacali
Le Profondità della Quiete

Lettura dei Tarocchi
Lord Shiva
Massaggio Olistico
Menando Il Can Per L'Aia
Morto Che Cammina
Notiziario Reiki
Perle di Saggezza
Risposte per l'Anima
Semi di Illuminazione
Sovrappeso? No Problem!
Transizione Vegetariana
Viaggio nel Mondo di Sotto
Zen Il Senso del Non Senso

Thank You For Reading
Managing Climate Change Consequences
Dr. Andrea Scarsi

www.ingramcontent.com/pod-product-compliance
Lightning Source LLC
Chambersburg PA
CBHW072337270726
48659CB00022B/1769